CW00504529

Keto Chaffles for your Breakfast

50 Quick and Creative Easy Chaffle Recipes to Make for All Occasions

Michelle Sells

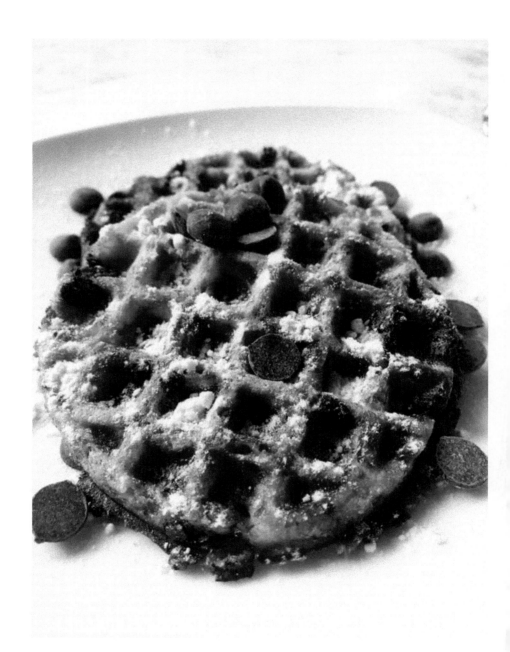

© Copyright 2021 - All rights reserved.

The content contained within this book may not be reproduced, duplicated or transmitted without direct written permission from the author or the publisher.

Under no circumstances will any blame or legal responsibility be held against the publisher, or author, for any damages, reparation, or monetary loss due to the information contained within this book. Either directly or indirectly.

Legal Notice:

This book is copyright protected. This book is only for personal use. You cannot amend, distribute, sell, use, quote or paraphrase any part, or the content within this book, without the consent of the author or publisher.

Disclaimer Notice:

Please note the information contained within this document is for educational and entertainment purposes only. All effort has been executed to present accurate, up to date, and reliable, complete information. No warranties of any kind are declared or implied. Readers acknowledge that the author is not engaging in the rendering of legal, financial, medical or professional advice. The content within this book has been derived from various sources. Please consult a licensed professional before attempting any techniques outlined in this book.

By reading this document, the reader agrees that under no circumstances is the author responsible for any losses, direct or indirect, which are incurred as a result of the use of information contained within this document, including, but not limited to, — errors, omissions, or inaccuracies.

Table of Contents

50 Essential Chaffle Recipes

1 Peanut Butter Keto Chaffle Cake

Preparation Time: 5 minutes

Cooking Time: 10 minutes

Servings: 2

Ingredients:

- For Chaffles:
- Egg: 1
- Peanut Butter:: 2 tbsp (sugar-free)
- Monkfruit: 2 tbsp
- Baking powder: ¼ tsp
- Peanut butter extract: ¼ tsp
- Heavy whipping cream: 1 tsp
- For Peanut Butter Frosting:
- Monkfruit: 2 tsp

- Cream cheese: 2 tbsp
- Butter: 1 tbsp
- Peanut butter: 1 tbsp (sugar-free)
- Vanilla: ¼ tsp

Directions:

1. Preheat a mini waffle maker if needed and grease it
2. In a mixing bowl, beat eggs and add all the chaffle ingredients
3. Mix them all well and pour the mixture to the lower plate of the waffle maker
4. Close the lid
5. Cook for at least 4 minutes to get the desired crunch
6. Remove the chaffle from the heat and keep aside for around a few minutes
7. Make as many chaffles as your mixture and waffle maker allow
8. In a separate bowl, add all the frosting ingredients and whisk well to give it a uniform consistency

9. Assemble chaffles in a way that in between two chaffles you put the frosting and make the cake

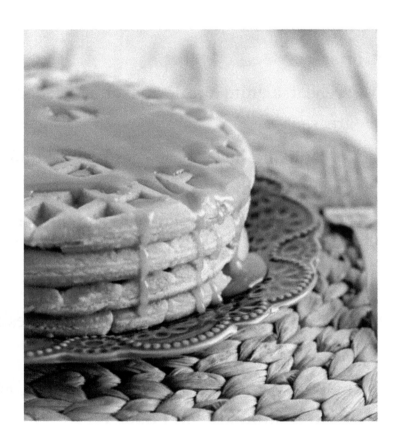

2 Strawberry Shortcake Chaffle

Preparation Time: 5 minutes

Cooking Time: 10 minutes

Servings: 2

Ingredients:

- Egg: 1

- Heavy Whipping Cream: 1 tbsp

- Any non-sugar sweetener: 2 tbsp

- Coconut Flour: 1 tsp

- Cake batter extract: ½ tsp

- Baking powder: ¼ tsp

- Strawberry: 4 or as per your taste

Directions:

1. Preheat a mini waffle maker if needed and grease it

2. In a mixing bowl, beat eggs and add non-sugar sweetener, coconut flour, baking powder, and cake batter extract

3. Mix them all well and pour the mixture to the lower plate of the waffle maker

4. Close the lid

5. Cook for at least 4 minutes to get the desired crunch

6. Remove the chaffle from the heat and keep aside for around two minutes

7. Make as many chaffles as your mixture and waffle maker allow

8. Serve with whipped cream and strawberries on top

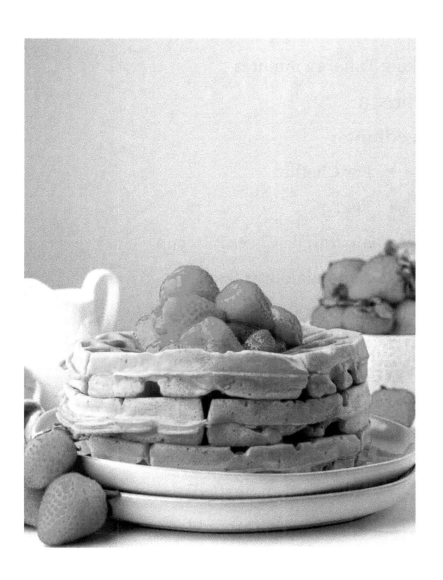

3 Italian Cream Chaffle Cake

Preparation Time: 8 minutes

Cooking Time: 12 minutes

Servings: 3

Ingredients:

- For Chaffle:
- Egg: 4
- Mozzarella Cheese: ½ cup
- Almond flour: 1 tbsp
- Coconut flour: 4 tbsp
- Monkfruit sweetener: 1 tbsp
- Vanilla extract: 1 tsp
- Baking powder: 1 ½ tsp
- Cinnamon powder: ½ tsp
- Butter: 1 tbsp (melted)
- Coconut: 1 tsp (shredded)
- Walnuts: 1 tsp (chopped)
- For Italian Cream Frosting:

- Cream cheese: 4 tbsp
- Butter: 2 tbsp
- Vanilla: ½ tsp
- Monkfruit sweetener: 2 tbs

Directions:

1. Blend eggs, cream cheese, sweetener, vanilla, coconut flour, melted butter, almond flour, and baking powder
2. Make the mixture creamy
3. Preheat a mini waffle maker if needed and grease it
4. Pour the mixture to the lower plate of the waffle maker
5. Close the lid
6. Cook for at least 4 minutes to get the desired crunch
7. Remove the chaffle from the heat and keep aside to cool it
8. Make as many chaffles as your mixture and waffle maker allow

9. Garnish with shredded coconut and chopped walnuts

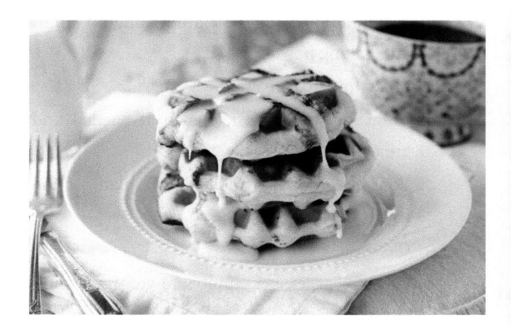

4 Banana Cake Pudding Chaffle

Preparation Time: 10 minutes

Cooking Time: 1 hour

Servings: 2

Ingredients:

- For Banana Chaffle:
- Cream cheese: 2 tbsp
- Banana extract: 1 tsp
- Mozzarella cheese: ¼ cup
- Egg: 1
- Sweetener: 2 tbsp
- Almond flour: 4 tbsp
- Baking powder: 1 tsp
- For Banana Pudding:
- Egg yolk: 1 large
- Powdered sweetener: 3 tbsp
- Xanthan gum: ½ tsp
- Heavy whipping cream: 1/2 cup

- Banana extract: ½ tsp
- <u>Salt: a pinch</u>

Directions:

1. In a pan, add powdered sweetener, heavy cream, and egg yolk and whisk continuously so the mixture thickens

2. Simmer for a minute only

3. Add xanthan gum to the mixture and whisk again

4. Remove the pan from heat and add banana extract and salt and mix them all well

5. Shift the mixture to a glass dish and refrigerate the pudding

6. Preheat a mini waffle maker if needed and grease it

7. In a mixing bowl, add all the chaffle ingredients

8. Mix them all well and pour the mixture to the lower plate of the waffle maker

9. Close the lid

10. Cook for at least 5 minutes to get the desired crunch

11. Remove the chaffle from the heat and keep aside for around a few minutes

12. Stack chaffles and pudding one by one to form a cake

5 Cream Coconut Chaffle Cake

Preparation Time: 20 minutes

Cooking Time: 1 hour 20 minutes (depends on your refrigerator)

Servings: 2

Ingredients:

- For Chaffles:
- Egg: 2
- Powdered sweetener: 2 tbsp
- Cream cheese: 2 tbsp
- Vanilla extract: 1/2 tsp
- Butter: 1 tbsp (melted)
- Coconut: 2 tbsp (shredded)
- Coconut extract: ½ tsp
- For Filling:
- Coconut: ¼ cup (shredded)
- Butter: 2 tsp
- Monkfruit sweetener: 2 tbsp
- Xanthan gum: ¼ tsp

- Salt: a pinch
- Egg yolks: 2
- Almond: 1/3 cup unsweetened
- Coconut milk: 1/3 cup
- For Garnishing:
- Whipped Cream: as per your taste
- Coconut: 1 tbsp (shredded)

Directions:

1. Preheat a mini waffle maker if needed and grease it
2. In a mixing bowl, add all the chaffle ingredients
3. Mix them all well and pour the mixture to the lower plate of the waffle maker
4. Close the lid
5. Cook for at least 4 minutes to get the desired crunch
6. Remove the chaffle from the heat and keep aside for around a few minutes
7. Make as many chaffles as your mixture and waffle maker allow

8. For the filling, in a small pan, cook almond milk and coconut together on medium heat in such way that it only steams but doesn't boil

9. In another bowl, lightly whish egg yolks and add milk to it continuously

10. Heat the mixture so it thickens, again it must not boil

11. Add sweetener and whisk while adding Xanthan Gum bit by bit

12. Remove from heat and mix all the other ingredients

13. Mix well and refrigerate; the mixture will further thicken when cool

14. Assemble the prepared chaffles and cream on top of one another to make the cake-like shape

15. Garnish with coconuts and whipped cream at the end

6 Lemon Chaffle Cake

Preparation Time: 40 minutes (depends on chaffle's cooling)

Cooking Time: 20 minutes

Servings: 2

Ingredients:

- For Chaffles:
- Egg: 2
- Powdered sweetener: 1 tbsp
- Cream cheese: 4 tbsp
- Butter: 2 tbsp (melted)
- Coconut flour: 2 tsp
- Baking powder: 1 tsp
- Lemon extract: ½ tsp
- Cake batter extract: 20 drops
- For Frosting:
- Heavy whipping cream: ½ cup
- Monkfruit sweetener: 1 tbsp
- Lemon extract: ¼ tsp

Directions:

1. Preheat a mini waffle maker if needed and grease it

2. In a blender, add all the chaffle ingredients and blend

3. Pour the mixture to the lower plate of the waffle maker and spread it evenly to cover the plate properly

4. Close the lid

5. Cook for at least 4 minutes to get the desired crunch

6. Remove the chaffle from the heat and keep aside

7. Make as many chaffles as your mixture and waffle maker allow

8. Prepare the frosting by whisking all the frosting ingredients till it thickens and attains uniform consistency

9. When all the chaffles cool down, arrange in the form of cake by adding frosting in between

7 Keto Birthday Chaffle Cake

Preparation Time: 40 minutes

Cooking Time: 20 minutes

Servings: 2

Ingredients:

- For Chaffle:
- Egg: 2
- Powdered sweetener: 2 tbsp
- Cream cheese: 2 tbsp
- Butter: 2 tbsp (melted)
- Coconut flour: 2 tsp
- Almond flour: ¼ cup
- Baking powder: ½ tsp
- Vanilla extract: ½ tsp
- Xanthan powder ¼ tsp
- For Frosting:
- Heavy whipping cream: 1/2 cup
- Swerve: 2 tbsp

- Vanilla extract: ½ tsp

Directions:

1. Preheat a mini waffle maker if needed

2. In a medium-size blender, add all the cake ingredients and blend till it forms a creamy texture

3. Let the batter sit for a minute or two; appearance is watery but it produces crunchy chaffles

4. Pour the batter to the lower plate of the waffle maker and spread it evenly to cover the plate properly

5. Close the lid

6. Cook for at least 4 minutes to get the desired crunch

7. Remove the chaffle from the heat and keep aside to cool totally

8. For the frosting, add all the ingredients in a bowl and use a hand mixer until the cream thickens

9. Make as many chaffles as your mixture and waffle maker allow

10. Frost the chaffles in a way you like

11. Serve cool and enjoy!

8 Tiramasu Chaffle Cake:

Preparation Time: 20 minutes

Cooking Time: 40 minutes

Servings: 4

Ingredients:

- Egg: 2
- Monkfruit sweetener: 2 tbsp
- Cream cheese: 2 tbsp
- Butter: 2 tbsp (melted)
- Coconut flour: 2 tbsp
- Baking powder: 1 tsp
- Vanilla extract: ½ tsp
- Instant coffee dry mix: 2 ½ tsp
- Hazelnut extract: ½ tsp
- Almond flour: ¼ cup
- Organic cacao powder: 1 ½ tbsp
- Himalayan pink fine salt: 1/8 tsp
- Mascarpone Cheese: ½ cup

- Powdered sweetener: ¼ cup

Directions:

1. In a microwave, melt butter for a minute and then add instant coffee, stir it continuously
2. In a bowl, beat eggs, cream cheese and the butter-coffee mixture
3. In a separate bowl, add sweetener, vanilla extract, and mascarpone cheese
4. In the egg mixture, add all the dry ingredients into it and mix well
5. Preheat a mini waffle maker if needed and grease it
6. Pour the egg mixture to the lower plate of the waffle maker and spread it evenly to cover the plate properly and close the lid
7. Cook for at least 4 minutes to get the desired crunch
8. Remove the chaffle from the heat and keep aside to cool down
9. Make as many chaffles as your mixture and waffle maker allow

10. If you want to have two layers cake then split the cream

11. You can also separate cacao powder ½ tbsp and instant coffee ½ tsp and blend

12. Layer the cake in a way that spread cream and coffee mixture on one chaffle and add another chaffle on top

13. Serve cool and enjoy!

9 Birthday Cake Chaffle

Preparation time: 10 minutes

Cooking time: 12 minutes

Servings: 2

Ingredients:

- 1 egg (beaten)
- 2 tbsp almond flour
- 1 tbsp swerve sweetener
- ½ tsp cake batter extract
- ¼ tsp baking powder
- 1 tbsp heavy whipping cream
- 2 tbsp cream cheese
- ½ tsp vanilla extract
- ½ tsp cinnamon
- Frosting:
- 1 tbsp swerve
- ¼ cup heavy whipping cream
- ½ tsp vanilla extract

Directions:

1. Plug the waffle maker to preheat it and spray it with a non-stick spray.

2. In a mixing bowl, combine the cinnamon, almond flour, baking powder and swerve.

3. In another mixing bowl, whisk together the egg, vanilla, heavy cream, and cake batter extract.

4. Pour the flour mixture into the egg mixture and mix until the ingredients are well combined and you have formed a smooth batter.

5. Pour an appropriate amount of the batter into the waffle maker and spread out the waffle maker to cover all the holes on the waffle maker.

6. Close the waffle maker and bake for about 3 minutes or according to your waffle maker's settings.

7. After the cooking cycle, use a silicone or plastic utensil to remove the chaffle from the waffle maker.

8. Repeat step 5 to 7 until you have cooked all the batter into chaffles.

9. For the cream, whisk together the swerve, heavy cream and vanilla extract until smooth and fluffy.

10.   To assemble the cake, place one chaffle on a flat surface and spread 1/3 of the cream over it. Layer another chaffle on the first one and spread 1/3 of the cream over it too. Repeat this for the last chaffle and the remaining cream.

Cut cake and serve.

10 Chocolate Chaffle Cake

Preparation Time: 2 minutes

Cooking Time: 8 minutes

Servings: 2

Ingredients

- 2 tablespoons cocoa powder
- 2 tablespoons swerve granulated sugar
- 1 egg
- 1 tablespoon overwhelming whipping cream
- 1 tablespoon almond flour
- 1/4 tsp preparing powder
- 1/2 tsp vanilla concentrate

Directions:

1. Add all the recipes together to get the exact formula

11 Keto Blueberry Waffles

Preparation Time: 3 minutes

Cooking Time: 15 minutes

Servings: 5

Ingredients

- 1 cup of mozzarella cheddar
- 2 tablespoons almond flour
- 1 tsp heating powder
- 2 eggs
- 1 tsp cinnamon
- 2 tsp of Swerve
- 3 tablespoon blueberries

Directions

1. Heat up your Dash smaller than expected waffle producer.
2. In a blending, bowl includes the mozzarella cheddar, almond flour, heating powder, eggs, cinnamon, swerve and blueberries. Blend well so every one of the fixings is combined.

3. Spray your smaller than expected waffle producer with nonstick cooking shower.

4. Add shortly less than 1/4 a cup of blueberry keto waffle player.

5. Close the top and cook the chaffle for 3-5 minutes. Check it at the brief imprint to check whether it is firm and dark-colored. In the event that it isn't or it adheres to the highest point of the waffle machine close the cover and cook for 1-2 minutes longer.

6. Serve with a sprinkle of swerve confectioners sugar or keto syrup.

12 Keto Pizza Chaffle

Preparation time: 15 minutes

Cooking time: 6 minutes

Ingredients

- 1 tsp coconut flour
- 1 egg white
- 1/2 cup mozzarella cheddar, destroyed
- '1 tsp cream cheddar, mollified
- 1/4 tsp preparing powder
- 1/8 tsp Italian flavoring
- 1/8 tsp garlic powder
- pinch of salt
- 3 tsp low carb marinara sauce
- 1/2 cup mozzarella cheddar
- 6 pepperonis cut down the middle
- 1 tbsp parmesan cheddar, destroyed
- 1/4 tsp basil flavoring

Directions:

1. Preheat stove to 400 degrees. Turn waffle creator on or plug it in so it gets hot.

2. In a little bowl include coconut flour, egg white, mozzarella cheddar, relaxed cream cheddar, heating powder, garlic powder, Italian seasonings, and a spot of salt.

3. Pour 1/2 of the player in the waffle producer, close the top, and cook for 3-4 minutes or until chaffle arrives at desired doneness.

4. Carefully expel chaffle from the waffle creator, at that point adhere to similar guidelines to make the second chaffle.

5. Top each chaffle with tomato sauce (I utilized 1/2 tsp per), pepperoni, mozzarella cheddar, and parmesan cheddar.

6. Place in the broiler on a preparing sheet (or straight on the heating rack) on the first-rate of the stove for 5-6 minutes. At that point turn the broiler to cook so the cheddar starts to air pocket and dark-colored. Keep a nearby

eye as it can consume rapidly. I cooked my pizza chaffle for approx 1 min and 30 seconds.

7. Remove from stove and sprinkle basil on top.

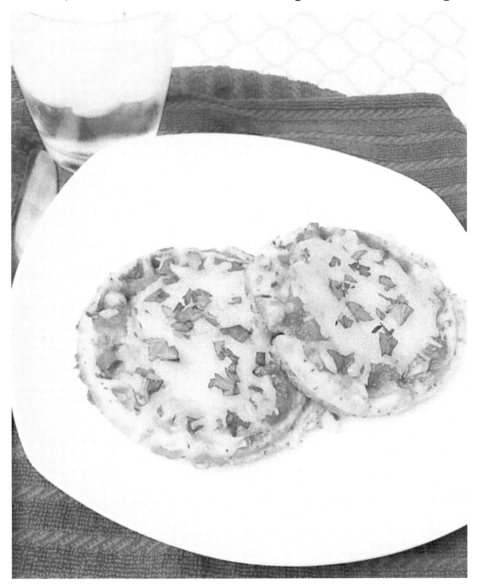

13 Traditional Keto Low Carb Chaffle

Preparation time: 10 minutes

Cooking time: 5 minutes

Ingredients:

- 1 egg

- 1/2 cup cheddar, destroyed

Directions

1. Turn waffle producer on or plug it in with the goal that it warms and oil the two sides.

2. In a little bowl, split an egg at that point include the 1/2 cup cheddar and mix to consolidate.

3. Pour 1/2 of the hitter in the waffle producer and close the top.

4. Cook for 3-4 minutes or until it arrives at wanted doneness.

5. Carefully expel from waffle producer and put in a safe spot for 2-3 minutes to give it an opportunity to fresh.

6. Follow the guidelines again to make the second chaffle.

7. This formula for a customary chaffle makes incredible sandwiches.

14 Essential Chaffle Recipe

Preparation time: 15 minutes

Cooking time: 5 minutes

Ingredients:

- 1/2 cup of cheddar, destroyed (you can utilize any cheddar)
- 1 egg
- 1 tsp of sans gluten preparing powder
- 2 tablespoons of almond flour (can substitute with 1 tablespoon of coconut flour whenever wanted)

Directions:

1. Assemble and set up the entirety of your fixings and preheat your waffle creator.
2. Combine your egg, destroyed cheddar, heating powder, and almond or coconut flour.
3. Empty a large portion of your blend into the waffle producer. Cook till done. Expel. Empty the rest of the hitter into the waffle producer and cook.

4. We purchased the little Dash brand small scale waffle producer and the lower than usual frying pan (you can utilize it is possible that one) to use with this formula and it makes the ideal size Chaffle. Try not to have a small scale waffle creator? You can utilize a standard waffle producer or skillet when necessary.

15 Lemon Delight Chaffle

Preparation time: 15 minutes

Cooking time: 0 minutes

Ingredients:

- 1 oz cream cheddar (mollified)
- 1/4 cup mozzarella cheddar, destroyed
- 1 egg
- 1 to 2 tsp lemon juice
- 2 tablespoons of sugar
- 1 tsp preparing powder
- 4 tablespoons of almond flour

Directions:

1. Add all the recipes together to get the exact formula!!!
2. Banana Nut Muffin Chaffle
3. 1 oz cream cheddar (mollified)
4. 1/4 cup mozzarella cheddar, destroyed
5. 1 egg
6. 1 tsp banana extricate

43

7. 2 tablespoons of sugar

8. 1 tsp preparing powder

9. 4 tablespoons of almond flour

10. 2 tablespoons of pecans or walnuts, hacked

Directions:

01. Add all the recipes together to get the exact formula!!!

16 McGriddle Chaffle

Preparation time: 15 minutes

Cooking time: 0 minutes

Ingredients:

1. 1 egg
2. 1 oz cream cheddar, relaxed
3. 1 tsp sugar
4. 1 tsp vanilla
5. 1 tablespoon keto-accommodating maple syrup (We use Lakanto)
6. 1/4 cup mozzarella cheddar, destroyed
7. 1 tsp of heating powder
8. <u>4 tablespoons of almond flour</u>
9. <u>Directions:</u>
1. Add all the recipes together to get the exact formula!!!

17 Chocolate Dream Chaffle

Preparation time: 15 minutes

Cooking time: 0 minutes

Ingredients:

- 1 egg
- 1/4 cup of mozzarella cheddar
- 1 oz cream cheddar
- 2 tsp sugar
- 2 tablespoons cacao powder
- 1 tsp vanilla
- 4 Tbsp almond flour
- 1 tsp heating powder
- Red Velvet Chaffle
- 1 egg
- 1/4 cup of mozzarella cheddar
- 1 oz cream cheddar
- 2 tsp sugar
- 2 tablespoons cacao powder

- 1 tsp red velvet concentrate

- 4 Tbsp almond flour

- 1 tsp preparing powder

Directions:

1. Add all the recipes together to get the exact formula!!!

18 Keto Italian Cream Chaffle Cake

Preparation time: 15 minutes

Cooking time: 10 minutes

Ingredients:

- Sweet Chaffle Ingredients:
- 4 oz Cream Cheese relaxed and room temp
- 4 eggs
- 1 tablespoon softened margarine
- 1 teaspoon vanilla concentrate
- 1/2 teaspoon cinnamon
- 1 tablespoon monk fruit sugar or your most loved keto-endorsed sugar
- 4 tablespoons coconut flour
- 1 tablespoon almond flour
- 1 1/2 teaspoons heating powder
- 1 tbs coconut destroyed and unsweetened
- 1 tbs pecans cleaved
- Italian Cream Frosting Ingredients:
- 2 oz cream cheddar mellowed and room temp

- 2 tbs margarine room temp

- 2 tbs monk fruit sugar or your most loved keto-endorsed sugar

- 1/2 teaspoon vanilla

Directions:

1. In a medium-size blender, include the cream cheddar, eggs, softened spread, vanilla, sugar, coconut flour, almond flour, and heating powder. Discretionary: Add the destroyed coconut and pecans to the blend or spare it for the icing. Whichever way is extraordinary!

2. Blend the fixings on high until it's smooth and rich.

3. Preheat the smaller than normal waffle creator.

4. Add the fixings to the preheated waffle creator.

5. Cook for around 2 to 3 minutes until the waffles are finished.

6. Remove and permit the chaffles to cool.

7. In a different bowl, begin to make the icing by including every one of the fixings together. Mix until it's smooth and rich.

8. Once the chaffles have totally cool, ice the cake.

9. Notes

10. Makes 8 smaller than expected chaffles or 3 to 4 huge chaffles

19 Easy Parmesan Chicken Chaffle

Preparation time: 10 minutes

Cooking time: 5 minutes

Ingredients

- Chaffle Ingredients:
- 1/2 cup canned chicken bosom
- 1/4 cup cheddar
- 1/8 cup parmesan cheddar
- 1 egg
- 1 tsp Italian flavoring
- 1/8 tsp garlic powder
- 1 tsp cream cheddar room temperature
- Besting Ingredients:
- 2 cuts of provolone cheddar
- 1 tbs sugar free pizza sauce

Directions

1. Preheat the small scale waffle creator.

2. In a medium-size bowl, include every one of the fixings and blend until it's completely joined.

3. Add a teaspoon of destroyed cheddar to the waffle iron for 30 seconds before including the blend. This will make the best outside layer and make it simpler to remove this overwhelming chaffle from the waffle creator when it's set.

4. Pour portion of the blend in the smaller than normal waffle producer and cook it for at least 4 to 5 minutes.

5. Repeat the above strides to cook the second Chicken Parmesan Chaffle.

6. Notes

7. Top with a sugar free pizza sauce and one cut of provolone cheddar. I like to sprinkle the top with much progressively Italian Seasoning as well!

20 Chickfila Copycat Chaffle Sandwich

Preparation time: 45 minutes

Cooking time: 25 minutes

Ingredients

- Elements for the Chicken:
- 1 Chicken Breast
- 4 T of Dill Pickle Juice
- 2 T Parmesan Cheese powdered
- 2 T Pork Rinds ground
- 1 T Flax Seed ground
- Salt and Pepper
- 2 T Butter dissolved
- Elements for Chaffle Sandwich Bun:
- 1 Egg room temperature
- 1 Cup Mozzarella Cheese destroyed
- 3 - 5 drops of Stevia Glycerite
- 1/4 tsp Butter Extract

Directions:

1. Directions for the Chicken:
2. Pound chicken to 1/2 inch thickness.
3. Cut down the middle and spot in zip lock baggie with pickle
4. Juice.
5. Seal baggie and spot in the cooler for 1 hour to medium-term.
6. Preheat Airfryer for 5 mins at 400
7. In a little shallow bowl, combine Parmesan cheddar, pork skins, flaxseed, and S&P.
8. Remove chicken from the baggie and dispose of pickle juice.
9. Dip chicken in dissolved margarine at that point in flavoring blend.
10.   Place material paper round in Airfryer container, brush the paper daintily with oil. (I utilized coconut)
11. Place chicken in preheated Airfryer and cook for 7 minutes.

12. Flip chicken and Airfry for an extra 7-8 mins. (This can change depending on the size of your check internal temp of 165*

13. Guidelines for Chaffle Bun:

14. Mix everything in a little bowl. Put 1/4 of the blend in the preheated small scale run waffle iron. Cook for 4 mins. Expel to a cooking rack. Rehash x3

15. Assemble Sandwich's: Place laid chicken on one Chaffle bun, includes 3 dill pickle cuts. Spread with different buns. Rehash.

16. Enjoy!

21 Banana Nut Chaffle

Preparation time: 15 minutes

Cooking time: 10 minutes

Ingredients

- 1 egg
- 1 tbs cream cheddar. mellowed and room temp
- 1 tbs sugar-free cheesecake pudding discretionary fixing since it is grimy keto
- 1/2 cup mozzarella cheddar
- 1 tbs Monkfruit confectioners
- 1/4 tsp vanilla concentrate
- 1/4 tsp banana remove
- Discretionary Toppings:
- Sugar-free caramel sauce
- Pecans

Directions

1. Preheat the smaller than normal waffle producer

2. In a little bowl, whip the egg.

3. Add the rest of the fixings to the egg blend and blend it until it's very much consolidated.

4. Add a large portion of the hitter to the waffle creator and cook it for at least 4 minutes until it's brilliant dark colored.

5. Remove the completed chaffle and include the other portion of the player to cook the other chaffle.

6. Top with your discretionary fixings and serve warm!

7. Notes

8. Top with your discretionary fixings and serve warm!

22 Pumpkin Chaffle with Cream Cheese Frosting

Preparation time: 15 minutes

Cooking time: 5 minutes

Ingredients

- 1 egg
- 1/2 cup mozzarella cheddar
- 1/2 tsp pumpkin pie zest
- 1 tbs pumpkin healthy pressed with no sugar included
- Optional Cream Cheese Frosting Ingredients:
- 2 tbs cream cheddar relaxed and room temperature
- 2 tbs monk fruit confectioners mix or any of your most loved keto-accommodating sugar
- 1/2 tsp clear vanilla concentrate

Directions

1. Preheat the smaller than expected waffle creator.

2. In a little bowl, whip the egg.

3. Add the cheddar, pumpkin pie zest, and the pumpkin.

4. Mix well.

5. Add 1/2 of the blend to the smaller than expected waffle creator and cook it for in any event 3 to 4 minutes until it's brilliant dark-colored.

6. While the chaffle is cooking, include the entirety of the cream cheddar icing fixings in a bowl and blend it until it's smooth and velvety.

7. Add the cream cheddar icing to the hot chaffle and serve it right away.

8. Notes

9. Add the cream cheddar icing to the hot chaffle and serve it right away

23 Crispy Everything Bagel Chaffle Chips

Preparation time: 20 minutes

Cooking time: 5 minutes

Ingredients

- 3 Tbs Parmesan Cheese destroyed
- 1 tsp Everything Bagel Seasoning

Directions

1. Preheat the smaller than expected waffle creator.

2. Place the Parmesan cheddar on the iron and enable it to bubble. Around 3 minutes. Make sure to leave it sufficiently long or else it won't turn firm when it cools. Significant advance!

3. Sprinkle the softened cheddar with around 1 teaspoon of Everything Bagel Seasoning. Leave the waffle iron open when it cooks!

4. Unplug the scaled-down waffle producer and enable it to cool for a couple of moments. This will allow the cheddar sufficiently cool to tie together and get fresh.

5. After around 2 minutes of it chilling, it will even now be warm.

6. Use a scaled-down spatula to strip the warm (however not hot cheddar from the smaller than usual waffle iron.

7. Allow it to cool totally for fresh chips! These chips pack an incredible crunch, which is something I will in general miss on Keto!

8. Notes

9. The more cheddar you utilize, the thicker the chips will be. The less cheddar you use the lighter and increasingly fresh the chips will be! This method functions admirably for the two surfaces! Make sure to use less Everything Bagel seasonings if you use less cheddar. You don't need the seasonings to be overwhelming to the proportion of cheddar you have

24 Keto BLT Chaffle Sandwich

Preparation time: 15 minutes

Cooking time: 5 minutes

Ingredients

- Chaffle bread fixings
- 1/2 cup mozzarella destroyed
- 1 egg
- 1 tbs green onion diced
- 1/2 tsp Italian flavoring
- Sandwich fixings
- Bacon pre-cooked
- Lettuce
- Tomato cut
- 1 tbs mayo

Directions:

1. Preheat the smaller than normal waffle creator

2. In a little bowl, whip the egg.

3. Add the cheddar, seasonings, and onion. Blend it until it's all around fused.

4. Place a large portion of the hitter in the smaller than usual waffle creator and cook it for 4 minutes.

5. If you need crunchy bread, include a tsp of destroyed cheddar to the smaller than normal waffle iron for 30 seconds before including the hitter. The additional cheddar outwardly makes the best covering!

6. After the first chaffle is finished, add the rest of the player to the smaller than usual waffle producer and cook it for 4 minutes.

7. Add the mayo, bacon, lettuce, and tomato to your sandwich.

25 Chocolate Chip Cookie Chaffle Cake

Preparation time: 15 minutes

Cooking time: 5 minutes

Ingredients

- Elements for cake layers:
- 1 T Butter liquefied
- 1 T Golden Monkfruit sugar
- 1 Egg Yolk
- 1/8 tsp Vanilla Extract
- 1/8 tsp Cake Batter Extract
- 3 T Almond Flour
- 1/8 tsp Baking Powder
- 1 T Chocolate Chips sugar-free
- Whipped Cream Frosting Ingredients:
- 1 tsp unflavored gelatin
- 4 tsp Cold Water
- 1 Cup HWC

- 2 T Confectioners Sweetener

Directions

1. Chocolate Chip Cookie Chaffle Cake Recipe Instructions
2. Cake Instructions
3. Mix everything and cook in a smaller than normal waffle iron for 4 mins. Rehash for each layer. I decided to make 3.
4. Whipped Cream Frosting Instructions
5. Place your mixers and your blending bowl in the cooler for around 15 minutes to enable them to cool.
6. In a microwave-safe bowl, sprinkle the gelatin over the virus water. Mix, and permit to "blossom". This takes around 5 minutes.
7. Microwave the gelatin blend for 10 seconds. It will end up being a fluid. Mix to ensure everything is broken down.
8. In your chilled blending bowl, start whipping the cream on a low speed. Include the confectioner's sugar.

9. Move to a higher speed and watch for good tops to start to the frame.

10. Once the whipping cream is beginning to top, switch back to a lower speed and gradually sprinkle the dissolved fluid gelatin blend in. When it's in, turn back to a higher speed and keep on beating until it's arrived at hardened pinnacles.

11. Place in channeling sacks and funnel on your cake.

12. Notes

13. I just utilized 1/2 of the whipped cream for this recipe.

26 Chaffle With Cranberry Purree

Preparation Time: 5 min

Cooking Time: 5 min

Servings: 4

Ingredients

- 2 large eggs
- 1/4 cup almond flour
- 3/4 tsp baking powder
- 1 cup mozzarella cheese, shredded
- Cooking spray
- ¼ cup cranberry puree cranberries for topping

Directions

1. Preheat your waffle maker according to manufacture instructions and grease with cooking spray.
2. Crack eggs in bowl and beat with almond flour and baking powder in mixing bowl.

3. Sprinkle half of cheese batter in waffle machine and pour half of egg batter over it.

4. Close chaffle machine and cook for 2-3 minutes.

5. Once cooked remove from maker.

6. Repeat with remaining batter

7. Pour cranberry puree and cranberries over it.

8. Serve with keto coffee and enjoy!

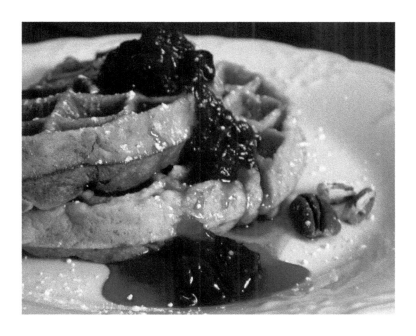

27 Basic Chaffles Recipe For Sandwiches

Preparation Time: 5 min

Cooking Time: 5 min

Servings: 2

Ingredients

- 1/2 cup mozzarella cheese, shredded
- 1 large egg
- 2 tbsps. almond flour
- 1/2 tsp psyllium husk powder
- 1/4 tsp baking powder
- 1 tsp stevia

Directions

1. Switch on and grease your waffle maker waffle maker with cooking spray.
2. Beat egg, cheese, almond flour, husk powder and baking powder.
3. Pour batter in the middle of waffle maker and close the lid.

4. Cook chaffles for about 2-3 minutes until cooked and light brown in color.

5. Carefully transfer chaffles to plate.

6. Serve with strawberry slice.

7. Enjoy!

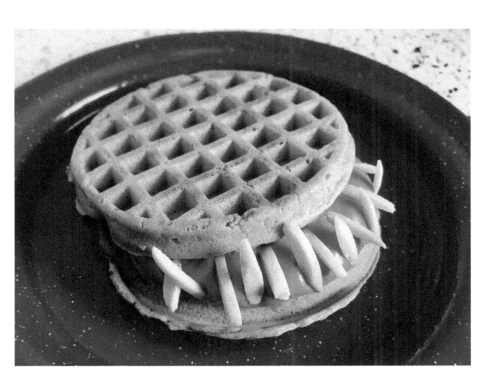

28 Savory Garlic Parmesan Chaffles

Preparation Time: 5 min

Cooking Time: 5 min

Servings: 4

Ingredients

- 1/2 cup cheddar cheese, shredded
- 1/3 cup parmesan cheese
- 1 large egg
- ½ tbsp. garlic powder
- 1/2 tsp onion powder
- 1/4 tsp baking powder
- <u>1 pinch salt</u>

Directions

1. Switch on your waffle maker and lightly grease your waffle maker with cooking spray.
2. Beat egg with garlic powder, onion powder, salt and baking powder in small mixing bowl.
3. Sprinkle ½ both cheese on waffle maker

4. Pour half of the egg batter into the middle of your waffle iron and close the lid.

5. Cook chaffles for about 2-3 minutes until crispy.

6. Once cooked remove chaffles from maker.

7. Drizzle garlic powder on top and enjoy!

29 Almond Flour Chaffles

Preparation Time: 5 min

Cooking Time: 5 min

Servings: 2

Ingredients

- 1 large egg
- 3/4 cup cheddar cheese, shredded
- 2 tbsps. almond flour
- 2 tbsps. cream cheese
- 1 tsp. stevia
- 1/2 tsp cinnamon powder
- 1/2 tsp vanilla extract
- 1/2 tsp psyllium husk powder
- 1/4 tsp baking powder

Directions

1. Switch on your waffle maker.
2. Grease your waffle maker with cooking spray and heat up on medium.

3. In a mixing bowl, beat egg with coconut flour, oil, stevia, cinnamon powder, vanilla, husk powder and baking powder.

4. Once egg is beaten well, add in cheese and mix again.

5. Pour half of the waffle batter into the middle of your waffle iron and close the lid.

6. Cook chaffles for about 2-3 minutes until crispy.

7. Serve with keto hot chocolate and enjoy!

30 Pumpkin Chaffles with Strawberries

Preparation Time: 5 min

Cooking Time: 5 min

Servings: 2

Ingredients

- 1/2 oz. cream cheese
- 1 large egg
- 1/2 cup mozzarella cheese, shredded
- 1 tsp. stevia
- 3 tsps. almond flour
- 1/2 tbsps. pumpkin pie spice
- 1/2 tsp vanilla extract
- 1/4 tsp baking powder

Directi ons

1. Grease your Belgian waffle maker with cooking spray and switch on.

2. Crack eggs in mixing bowl and with coconut flour, pumpkin spice, stevia, pumpkin spice, vanilla extract and baking powder.

3. Once ingredients are mix together with egg add in cheese and mix again.

4. Pour half of the chaffles batter into the middle of your waffle iron and close the lid.

5. Cook chaffles for about 2-3 until cooked and light golden.

6. Repeat with remaining batter

7. Once chaffles are cooked remove from maker.

8. Serve with BLT coffee and enjoy!

31 Spicy Jalapeno & Tomato Chaffle

Preparation Time: 5 min

Cooking Time: 5 min

Servings: 2

Ingredients

- 1 oz. cream cheese
- 1 large egg
- 1 pinch salt
- 1/2 cup cheddar cheese
- 1 tomato chopped
- 1 jalapenos chopped
- 1/4 tsp baking powder

Directions

1. Switch on your waffle maker and grease with cooking spray and let it preheat.
2. Beat egg with salt, baking powder and cream cheese in bowl.

3. Sprinkle chop tomato, jalapeno and cheese in waffle maker.

4. Pour egg mixture over cheese, close waffle maker.

5. Cook the chaffles for about 2-3 minutes until brown.

6. Once chaffles are cooked remove from maker.

7. Serve hot and enjoy!

32 Strawberries Purre Chaffles

Preparation Time: 5 min

Cooking Time: 5 min

Servings: 2

Ingredients

- 1 egg
- 1 cup mozzarella cheese, shredded
- 1 tbsp. almond flour
- 1/4 cup strawberry puree
- 1 tbsp. coconut flour for topping
- <u>Berries for topping</u>

Directions

1. Preheat your waffle maker as per the manufacturer instructions.
2. Grease your waffle maker with coconut oil.
3. Mix together egg, almond flour, and strawberry purée.
4. Add cheese and mix until well combined.

5. Pour batter in preheated and greased waffle maker and close the lid.

6. Cook strawberry chaffles for about 3-4 minutes or until cooked through.

7. Once cooked remove from maker

8. Drizzle coconut flour and berries on top.

9. Enjoy!

33 Simple Keto Cocoa Chaffles

Preparation Time: 5 min

Cooking Time: 5 min

Servings: 2

Ingredients

- 1 large egg

- 1/2 cup shredded mozzarella cheese

- 1 tbsp. cocoa powder

- <u>2 tbsps. almond flour</u>

Directions

1. Preheat your round waffle maker on medium high heat.

2. Mix together egg, cheese, almond flour, cocoa powder and vanilla in small mixing bowl.

3. Pour chaffles mixture into the center of the waffle iron.

4. Close the waffle maker and let cook for 3-5 minutes or until waffle is golden brown and set.

5. Carefully remove chaffles from the waffle maker.

6. Serve hot and enjoy!

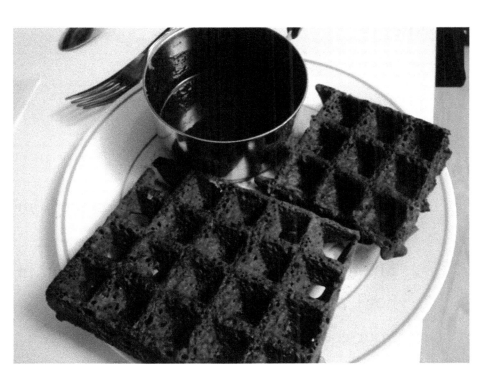

34 Simple Crispy Coconut Chaffle

Preparation Time: 5 min

ooking Time: 5 min

Servings: 2

Ingredients

- 1 large egg

- 1/2 cup shredded mozzarella cheese

- 2 tbsps. coconut flour

Directions

1. Preheat your square waffle maker on medium high heat.

2. Mix together egg, cheese and coconut flour in bowl.

3. Pour coconut chaffle batter in greased waffle maker.

4. Cook chaffles for 2-3 minutes or until cooked.

5. Once chaffle are cooked carefully removed from make.

6. Drizzle coconut flour and keto melted chocolate over it.

7. Serve hot and enjoy!

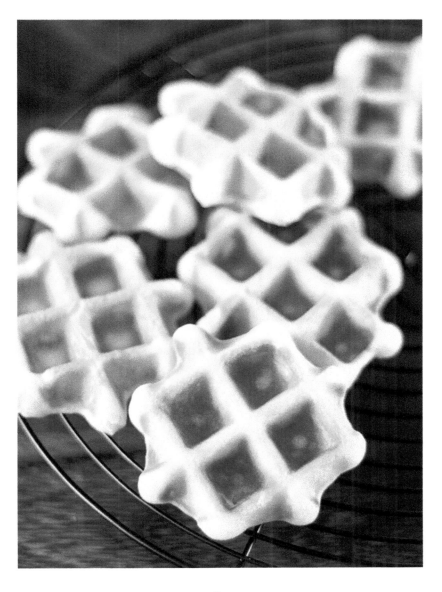

35 Morning Ham Chaffles Sandwich

Preparation Time: 5 min

Cooking Time: 5 min

Servings: 4

Ingredients

- 1 cup egg whites
- 1 cup cheddar cheese shredded
- ¼ cup almond flour
- ¼ cup heavy cream
- Topping
- 2 tomatoes, slice
- 4 ham slice
- 1 cucumber, sliced
- 1 scramble egg

Directions

1. Preheat your square waffle maker and grease with cooking spray.
2. Beat egg white in small bowl with flour.

3. Add shredded cheese in egg whites and mix well.

4. Add cream and cheese in egg mixture.

5. Pour Chaffles batter in waffle maker and close the lid.

6. Cook chaffles for about 4 minutes until crispy and brown.

7. Carefully remove chaffles from maker.

8. Serve with ham slice, scramble egg, tomato slice, cucumber slice.

01. Enjoy!

36 Brunch Chaffle Bowl

Preparation Time: 5 min

Cooking Time: 10 min

Srvings: 2

Ingredients

- 1/2 cup cheddar cheese
- 1/2 tsp. baking powder
- 1/4 cup egg whites
- Serving
- 1 egg fried
- 4 slice bacon
- salt and pepper to taste
- 1 tsp. avocado oil
- Berries for topping
- <u>Keto chocolate sauce</u>

Directions

1. Mix together all ingredients in a bowl.
2. Allow batter to sit while waffle iron warms.

3. Spray waffle iron with nonstick cooking spray.
4. Pour batter in waffle maker and cook according to directions of manufacturer.
5. Meanwhile heat oil in pan and fry bacon for 4-5 minutes until crispy. transfer cooked bacon in another plate.
6. Fry egg in same pan according to your choice.
7. Serve chaffles with berries, bacon, chocolate sauce and fried egg.
8. Enjoy!

37 Bacon Chaffles With Egg & Asparagus

Preparation Time: 5 min

Cooking Time: 10 min

Servings: 1

Ingredients

- 1 egg
- 1/4 cup cheddar cheese
- 2 tbsps. almond flour
- ½ tsp. baking powder
- 1 bacon slice, cooked
- TOPPING
- 1 egg
- 4-5 stalks asparagus
- 1 tsp avocado oil

Directions

1. Preheat waffle maker to medium high heat.
2. Mix chaffle ingredients in bowl except bacon.

3. Sprinkle cooked chopped bacon slice over waffle maker.

4. Spoon chaffles batter into the center of the waffle iron and cook for 2-3 minutes.

5. Meanwhile Sautee asparagus in heated oil and poach egg in boil water.

6. Once Chaffles are cooked remove from maker.

7. Serve chaffles with poach egg and asparagus

38 Coconut Chaffles With Boil Egg

Preparation Time: 5 min

Cooking Time: 5 min

Servings: 2

Ingredients

- 1 egg
- 1 oz. cream cheese,
- 1 oz. cheddar cheese
- 2 tbsps. coconut flour
- 1 tsp. stevia
- <u>1 egg, soft boil for serving</u>

Directions

1. Heat you mini Dash waffle maker and grease with cooking spray.
2. Mix together all chaffles ingredients in bowl.
3. Pour chaffle batter in preheated waffle maker.
4. Close the lid.
5. Cook chaffles for about 2-3 minutes until golden brown.

6. Serve with boil egg an enjoy!

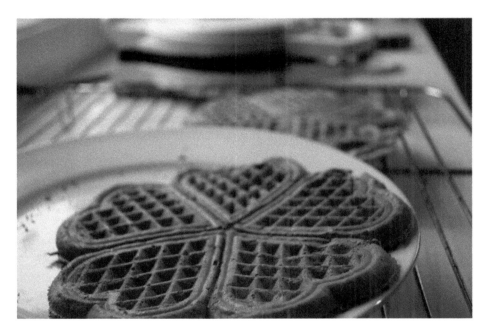

39 Chaffle With Parmeson

Preparation Time: 5 min

Cooking Time: 10 min

Servings: 1

Ingredients

- 1 egg

- 1/4 cup shredded cheddar cheese

- 2 tbsps. almond flour

- 1 tsp Italian seasoning

- ¼ cup parmesan cheese for topping

Direction s

1. Mix together egg cheese, almond flour and seasoning in bowl.

2. Switch on and grease waffle maker with cooking spray.

3. Pour batter in preheated waffle maker.

4. Cook chaffles for about 2-3 minutes until the chaffle is cooked through.

5. Meanwhile fry egg in non-stick pan for about 1-2 minutes.

6. For serving set fried egg on chaffles with feta cheese and tomatoes slice

40 Chaffle With Herbs

Preparation Time: 10 min

Cooking Time: 5 min

Servings: 1

Ingredients

- 1 large egg
- 1/4 cup cheddar cheese, shredded
- 1 tbsp. almond flour
- ¼ tsp. baking powder
- ½ tsp. garlic powder
- 1 tbsp. minced parsley
- For Serving
- 1 poach egg
- 4 oz. smoked salmon

Directions

1. Preheat your dash mini waffle maker and let it heat up and grease with cooking spray.

2. Mix together egg, cheese, almond flour, baking powder, garlic powder, parsley to a mixing bowl until combined well.

3. Pour batter in dash mini waffle maker.

4. Close the lid.

5. Cook chaffles for about 2-3 minutes or until cooked or no soggy.

6. Serve chaffles in plate with smoked salmon and poach egg.

01. Enjoy!

41 Chaffle Taco With Raspberries

Preparation Time: 5 min

Cooking Time: 15 min

Servings: 1

Ingredients

- 1 egg
- 1/4 cup mozzarella cheese, shredded
- 1/4 cup cheddar cheese, shredded
- 1 tsp coconut flour
- 1/4 tsp baking powder
- 1/2 tsp stevia
- For Topping
- 4 oz. raspberries
- 2 tbsps. coconut flour
- 2 oz. raspberry puree

Directions

1. Switch on your round waffle maker and grease is with cooking spray.

2. Mix together all chaffle ingredients in bowl and beat with fork.

3. Cook round chaffle in greased chaffle maker.

4. Once cooked remove from maker and immediately roll over kitchen roller for 5 minutes.

5. Meanwhile coat raspberries with in sauce and set on chaffle taco.

6. Sprinkle coconut flour on top.

7. Enjoy chaffle taco as dessert!

42 Chaffle Sandwich With Chicken

Preparation Time: 5 min

Cooking Time: 15 min

Servings: 2

Ingredients

- 1 large egg
- 1 cup cheddar cheese, shredded
- 1 pinch salt
- 1 tsp. baking powder
- For Serving
- 1 chicken thigh
- salt
- pepper
- 1 tsp. garlic, minced
- I tsp avocado oil
- 1 cucumber sliced
- 4-5 lettuce leaves
- 1 tomato sliced

- <u>4 slice cheddar cheese.</u>

Directions

1. Heat Belgian waffle maker and grease with cooking spray.
2. Mix together chaffle ingredients and make two Belgian chaffles batter in skillet and cook for about 2-3 minutes.
3. Meanwhile heat oil in pan, over medium heat.
4. Coat chicken thigh with salt, pepper and garlic.
5. Cook coated thigh in oil for about 4-5 minutes until cooked through.
6. Transfer cooked on Belgian chaffle top with lettuce leaves, tomato slice, cucumber slice, and lettuce leaves.
7. Cover sandwich and drizzle flax seeds on top.
8. Serve and enjoy!

43 Nutritious Creamy Chaffles

Preparation time: 5 min

Cooking time: 4 min

Servings: 2

Ingredients

- Eggs – 2
- Mozzarella – 1 cup
- Cream cheese – 2 tablespoons
- Almond flour – 2 tablespoons
- Baking powder – ¾ tablespoons
- Water (optional) – 2 tablespoons

Directions

1. Pre-heat waffle iron
2. Put listed ingredients in some bowl and mix
3. Grease waffle iron slightly and cook the mixture in it till crisp

44 Crunchy Jalapeno Chaffles

Preparation time: 4 min

Cooking time: 4 min

Servings: 2

Ingredients

- Eggs – 2
- Cheddar cheese – 1 ½ cups
- Jalapeno pepper – 16 slices

Directions:

1. Preheat waffle maker
2. Mix eggs and ¾ cups of cheddar cheese in a bowl
3. Shred cheddar cheese on waffle maker plate
4. Pour mixture onto plate
5. Add cheese on top of mixture
6. Top up with 4 Jalapeno slices and cook till crunchy

45 Crispy Simple Chaffles

Preparation time: 5 min

Cooking time: 10 min

Servings: 2

Ingredients

- Cheddar cheese (shredded) – 1/3 cup

- Eggs – 1

- Baking powder – ¼ teaspoon

- Flaxseed (ground) – 1 teaspoon

- Parmesan cheese (shredded) – 1/3 cup

Directions:

1. Mix all ingredients except parmesan cheese in one bowl

2. Shred half parmesan cheese on waffle iron to grease plate

3. Pour mixture and top with remaining shredded parmesan cheese

4. Cook till crispy

46 Bacon Bite Chaffles

Preparation time: 5 min

Cooking time: 5 min

Servings: 2

Ingredients

- Bacon bites (as desired)
- Cheddar cheese – 1 ½ cups

Directions:

1. Pre-heat waffle iron
2. Mix all ingredients in one bowl
3. Lightly grease waffle iron
4. Pour mixture and cook till crisp

470. Eggplant Chaffles

Preparation time: 10 min

Cooking time: 10 min

Servings: 2

Ingredients

- Eggplant – 1 medium

- Eggs – 1
- (Cheddar cheese – 1 ½ cups

Directions:

1. Boil eggplant for 15 min then blend
2. Preheat waffle iron
3. Mix listed ingredients in one bowl
4. Grease waffle iron, pour mixture and cook till crisp

47 Bacon Cheese Chaffles

Preparation time: 10 min

Cooking time: 10 min

Servings: 2

Ingredients

- Swiss cheese (shredded) – ½ cup
- Jalapenos (diced)– 1
- Bacon pieces – 2
- Eggs – 1

Directions:

1. Pre-heat waffle iron and grease
2. Fry bacon pieces in a pan
3. Add shredded cheese, egg and jalapenos and mix together
4. Cook till crisp

48 Crunchy Bacon Chaffles

Preparation time: 5 min

Cooking time: 5 min

Servings: 2

Ingredients

- Cheddar – 1/3 cup
- Eggs – 1
- Flaxseed (ground) – 1 teaspoon
- Baking powder – ¼ teaspoon
- Bacon piece – 2 tablespoons
- Parmesan – 1/3 cup

Directions:

1. Cook bacon in pan
2. Add egg, cheddar cheese, flaxseed and baking powder then mix
3. Shred part of parmesan cheese in waffle iron and grease plate
4. Pour mixture and top with remaining parmesan cheese

5. Cook till crisp

473. Crunchy Pickle Chaffles

Preparation time: 5 min

Cooking time: 5 min

Servings: 2

Ingredients

- Mozzarella – ½ cup
- Eggs – 1
- Pork Panko bread crumbs – ½ cup
- Pickle juice – 1 tablespoon
- Pickle slices – 8

Directions:

1. Pre-heat waffle iron
2. Mix ingredients together and pour thin layer onto waffle iron
3. Add drained pickle slices
4. Top with remaining mixture and cook till crisp

49 Bacon and Egg Chaffles

Preparation time: 5 min

Cooking time: 5 min

Servings: 2

Ingredients

- For Chaffles
- Cheddar – 1 cup
- Eggs – 2
- For Sandwich
- American cheese – 2 slices
- Bacon pieces – 4
- Eggs – 2

Directions:

1. Pre-heat and grease waffle maker
2. Mix eggs and cheddar cheese together
3. Pour mixture onto waffle plate and cook till crunchy
4. Cook bacon pieces till crispy then dry then

5. Fry eggs and add them in between two chaffles alongside bacon and cheese slices

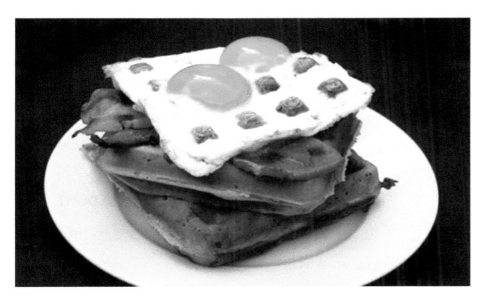

50 Almond Sandwich Chaffles

Preparation time: 5 min

Cooking time: 5 min

Servings: 2

Ingredients

- Cheddar cheese (shredded) – 1 cup
- Eggs – 2
- Almond flour – 2 tablespoons

Directions:

1. Pre-heat and grease waffle iron
2. Mix cheddar cheese and eggs in one bowl
3. Add the almond flour into mixture to enhance texture
4. Pour mixture onto waffle plate and cook till crunchy
5. Garnish ready and slightly cooled chaffles with preferred garnish
6. Takes 5 min to prepare and serves 2

Lightning Source UK Ltd.
Milton Keynes UK
UKHW020825170621
385666UK00005B/73